Anal fissure,

How to get rid of it naturally and fast

To everyone suffering from anal fissures!

Table of Contents

DISCLAIMER

This book is not intended to be a substitute for the medical recommendations of a doctor or other healthcare specialist. It's just a book to give some information for those suffering with anal fissures, and to help them cooperate with health specialists.

About writing this book

I took the initiative to write this book to share a remedy that can bring great relief to people living with anal fissures, to people we love and care about who are suffering from this terrible disease. Indeed, sharing knowledge is a duty or even a definite obligation, especially when we live in a community or a world where we advocate love, peace, harmony and development.

As for the disease, we all know that anal fissure is a very stressful disease. Yeah, you certainly know something about that! This disease is awful and very embarrassing. In fact, the first time you go to the toilet and feel intense pain and then see blood on the stool, it's worrying, it's even quite shocking internally. When this happens, you might think you have hemorrhoid diseases in the first place. It's hard and it's really disturbing and absolutely stressful. It's a disease that directly affects a person's sensitivity!

So far, following a particular experience, I waited weeks and weeks again for the wound to heal itself. But nothing was done so far! And when the crack started to get more and more unbearable, I went on the net to look for information about the symptoms. But after consulting with specialists, I realized that it was "the anal fissure" and not the hemorrhoid. It was already a small relief even though I knew that there was not yet a very effective treatment to cure this disease. However, I was able to keep hope and think about what I would do next. So I decided to go to the pharmacy for medication and advice. But, after a long period of treatments and nearly six months battling with this thing, the anal fissure, I never got any satisfactory results. Nothing was done, and the crack was still out there. It was really traumatic. I then began to lose hope, and a fear began to take hold, that fear or that feeling of being condemned to live with this disease for years ahead.

However, at some point, I came to my senses and thought that it would be okay; that there had to be a way to overcome this thing, that there would have to be a special or even a hidden cure! It was from there that I decided, through my own researches and investigations, to experiment with new things, things much more natural, new kinds of treatments with a "natural" product. I started thinking and meditating. It was so important to me, and I knew it would soon be a bad memory, especially a bad memory for that person who is dear to me and who was suffering from it. I knew how to help keep the hope! At one point, I thought of nature, of something natural.

In fact, we do live in a very rich environment, an environment where there are so many diseases that can be cured with the use of natural products. The anal fissure being an "external" disease, I knew there wouldn't be much risks or at least a major risk in trying something that I wouldn't say was new, but was still unknown to me. From that moment on, I thought of products that were miraculous to the skin, products that protect the skin without any risk of side effects. Then all I had to do was try, yes, and I knew it was safe. And it is in this way that I managed to get the anal fissure completely healed, and to finally get rid off the troubles and stress it was causing so far.

INTRODUCTION

Introduction

Anal fissure is probably one of the most embarrassing and troubling diseases that an individual can contract. It spares no one, and can so far affect younger people as well as older ones. But not all people are unfortunate enough to contract it in their lives. Yes, some people may have a chance of not experiencing this very embarrassing disease which is the anal fissure.

In principle anal fissure is not a very common disease, although it is devastating, and we hear about it almost any day. It is more likely to be related to discrete infections of which even the people it affects often do not dare to talk about it in public or with their relatives. In fact, it's because of that fact that anal fissure is not a very well-known disease to the public and it's only, most of the time, the people it directly affects who know about it. Anal fissures can also be ranked among the most traumatic diseases. Indeed, when you contract the anal fissure, most of the time you become stressed, traumatized, and in some cases, very wound up. We live with a daily trauma that even our family and friends often do not understand. It just becomes terrible moments for the person who suffers from it. We are always confronted with situations that are very difficult to manage and to live in. In fact, we always have our mind busy and this can cause us psychological problems. It is for these reasons that we must always be careful to quickly find ways to get rid of this traumatic disease which is the anal fissure as soon as possible.

Sometimes it is also important to consider that the first-time sight of blood stains in the feces can lead us think of having contracted hemorrhoids. Especially since this doubt is accentuated by the presence of blood in the excrements and the feeling of pain in the anus. Indeed, there are so many people who misunderstand the symptoms of anal fissures, and to whom when this happens for the first time to them, they confuse it with the symptoms of hemorrhoids. Yet it is important to know that anal fissure is quite different from hemorrhoid disease.

Chapter 1:

What is anal fissures?

Chapter 1: What is anal fissures?

An anal fissure, as its name suggests, is a small cracking on the anal canal wall. It's sort of a small lesion in the rectum. This low position on which the crack manifests itself makes it almost daily exposed to the painful effects of anal fissures. If we consider that a person should at least go to the stool once a day, then we can assume that people suffering from anal fissures are exposed at least once a day to the appalling experience of rectal pain.

In fact, the anal fissure is a small wound in the rectum. So, for it to heal quickly, it will need time to dry and be completely disinfected. However, the obligatory daily passage of stool at the anal canal level means that the wound is always wet and exposed to the germs contained in the stool. It is this repetitive situation on a daily basis that brings all the complexity to the process of healing the anal fissure, because whatever you might do, you will always find that the wound won't have time to dry and stay intact. Besides, this obligatory passage of the stool in this part of our body, and especially if the stool is hard, always reopens the wound at the level of the rectum: This is what brings bleeding.

The anal fissure manifests itself in acute pain at the time of bowel movements, accompanied by slight bleeding. It practically affects young people as well as adults, and does not even spare little babies. In fact, anal cracks are the first causes of bleeding in the rectal canal, which most often affect children. Some children are sometimes exposed as early as their infancy, especially those between 6 months and 2 years of age. This is what makes some babies untenable and spend all their time crying, and the most serious thing is that some parents realize it too late, because children at this age are often unable to speak. So be warned, as a parent, if you have a child who cries a lot, consult with them to see if they are not hurt anywhere on the body and have no cracks.

Unlike children, anal fissure in adults is often very quickly noticed and diagnosed. In some cases, it can happen that some people who have had this for the first time confuse it with a case of hemorrhoid or another disease of the type.

Anal fissure manifests itself in the form of bleeding in stool and burns in the rectum. When you contract an anal fissure, you will see blood stains on your stool every time you go to the toilet. You will have constant difficulty in bowel movements and you will always experience severe pain in the rectum as you relieve yourself. This pain also becomes much more unbearable when you have hard stools or if you get constipation. You will have constant pain in the rectum and in some cases, when you come back directly from the stool, you always feel this pain between your buttocks when you want to sit on a chair or sit somewhere else. And it is these constraints that make living with the anal fissure very painful and stressful.

Chapter 2:

Causes of an anal fissure

Chapter 2: Causes of an anal fissure

Anal fissures can be caused by several factors. But in most cases, frequent attacks of constipation or hard bowel issues are the main causes.

Anal cracks may be common in adults. The crack is often not of the same size or complication, so some cases may be more serious than others. Ultimately, it should be noted that anal cracks are often caused by:

- ❖ Hard stools : this is one of the most frequent causes. We all know the rectal canal is very sensitive. It is a zone narrow enough to allow the evacuation of stools smoothly. With hard stools, the rectal canal can easily be affected. Indeed it is never even comfortable when having hard stools, especially when suffering from constipation. The evacuation of stool always causes problems and the individual even feels pain in the anus. This sensation is already a sign that there is a problem, and that the area is tight. If you want to force or undergo the same practice repeatedly, there is a risk of exposing the rectal canal to crack. It is therefore advisable to consult a specialist if in case of constipation or if exposed to hard stool syndrome.

- ❖ By certain cases of inflammatory and chronic bowel diseases: Good bowel hygiene is vital to avoid certain types of bowel diseases or other rectal canal problems. Indeed, it is in the intestines that stools are stored, and it is from there that they are evacuated through the anus. Therefore, if an individual suffers from a chronic bowel disease, it can cause problems when going to the stool or cause bleeding. Anus inflammation can also cause these kinds of problems. It is important to get immediate treatment if you notice these types of anomalies.

❖ Frequent or repeated diarrhea: Diarrhea is the enemy of quietness! With diarrhea, it's always back and forth to the toilets. Since the rectal canal is sensitive, it becomes then exposed. Frequent cases of diarrhoea can cause inflammation of the anus. It is therefore important to consult a doctor immediately in case of diarrhoea.

❖ Anal sexual practice (such as sodomy) : The rectal canal is narrow, so with sodomy or other types of anal sex practices, it may be exposed. It is therefore important to be very careful.

Anal fissures can also affect us overnight because of some behavioral changes in the toilet. Indeed, some cases of anal cracks might have nothing to do with the causes listed above, but with certain types of bad behavior during or after bowel actions. We can cite some of them:

✦ Rushing or "Forcing": It can be ranked among the most frequent causes! Rushing in the stool is one of the best ways to get anal fissures. Sometimes you can have faeces that are not hard, but when trying to force them out, you end up cracking the rectal canal. That's why you have to take your time when you're in the saddle and relieve yourself easily, without forcing the process. So, take your time!

✦ Toilet paper: Using toilet paper improperly after relief can lead to infection in the rectum. The bottom of the rectum canal is very sensitive and should not be scratched or cleaned out by any means. Too much scrubbing with toilet paper can cause damage to the anus. Certain types of toilet paper are rigid, and can therefore cause injuries if pressed too hard on the anal tissue which is very sensitive. So, you have to take these details into account and pay attention to the use of toilet paper after bowel movements and be careful not to hurt the anus.

Chapter 3:

The Natural and Ideal Treatment to get rid of an Anal Fissure

Chapter 3: The natural and ideal treatment to get rid of an anal fissure

There are many possibilities for resolving anal fissures; however, results are not always guaranteed for some procedures and treatments. Indeed there are countless ideas and kinds of solutions on the market or on the internet concerning anal fissures. However, it is a fact that these "solutions" still do not provide "comfort" to the patient ; they generally do not help as a remedy.

From this perspective, we present a completely new natural method that can help you forget your daily nightmares about the symptoms of a terrible anal fissure.

As for the treatment of anal fissures, we experimented a very simple method with a natural product: it is the use of Shea butter!

How do you do that?

Practice is not difficult even if it requires discretion.

Simply use Shea butter!

Shea butter has extremely rare and very practical health benefits. It is a natural product very rich in vitamins. Nowadays, with Shea butter, we have the opportunity to treat anal fissures permanently!

To treat anal fissures, simply use Shea butter daily as a lubricant and whenever you go to the stool.

For the procedure:

1. Take your tube of Shea butter with you to the bathroom;

2. Before sitting on the chair, open the tube and take a pinch of Shea butter (about 3 grams);

3. Take the Shea butter portion on your finger (bring a large area with your finger)
   and apply it to your anus. With your finger, try to insert it through the rectum canal
   as much as possible, and until the tear wound is completely covered with butter.
   Play with your finger to dispense the gel, and make sure the channel is lubricated
   enough to ensure a smooth and soft passage of the stool.

4. After having introduced enough natural lubricant (Shea butter) you can now begin
   your relief.

Repeat the procedure every time you have to go for a bowel movement. In less than
three weeks, you will see the satisfying results.

So far, it is recommended to use natural Shea butter, which has never been diluted or
mixed with any other product.

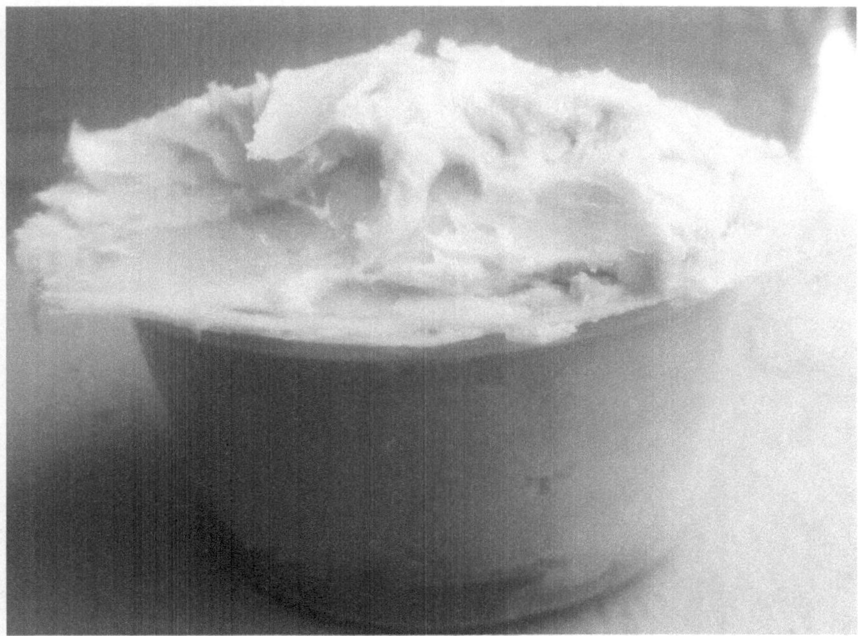

Picture of a box of Sea Butter

Shea butter has exceptional natural and sanitary qualities if it is very well preserved. It is a natural product with countless virtues. But, it is therefore very important that you carefully store the Shea butter in a healthy place.

What's really interesting about Shea butter is that it's a practically safe to use product with no particular side effects!

Biologically, the Shea butter is neutral and does not cause any allergic reaction, disease, poisoning or chemical burns. Its use does not cause any cases of intoxication or burns. It is just appropriate to carefully make a quality choice; avoid mixed products and use naturally pure butter, without mixing.

The rectum wall is naturally dry. But, with natural habits and needs, it is always exposed to germs. As a result, when having a crack and going to the stool, it becomes easy to get hurt again. In fact the bowel movement always causes the injury. Using Shea butter as a natural lubricant makes it easier to pass stools and to avoid always hurting the anus each time going to the stool.

NB: *For women, do not insert your finger directly into the vagina after inserting it into the rectum, as the anus contains germs that can cause fungal infections and other urinary tract infections. Wash your finger beforehand with water after inserting it into the rectum.*

Also, even after the rectal wound has healed, you can continue to use Shea butter before bowel movements; this will help prevent damage to the anus and allow for smooth bowel movement.

Chapter 4:

Top Virtues of Shea butter

Chapter 4: Top Virtues of Shea butter

Shea butter is a natural product that comes from the seeds of a Shea tree that grows in tropical Africa. It is an enriching product that can give a smooth and healthy skin.

Shea butter is full of some very important virtues and is naturally rich in vitamins A, E and F. It provides the skin with the necessary natural nutritional supplements and protects it from UV rays. It provides healthy skin, but also smooth hair.

Shea butter contains substances that nourish the skin, provides it with natural oils and helps fight against dry skin problems. It also allows the skin to produce collagen naturally.

Shea butter has also proven to be anti-inflammatory. It therefore helps to fight against skin inflammation and prevent certain skin infections.

In fact, Shea butter is a multi-purpose cream.

Here is a list of 11 reasons to start using Shea butter:

1. Nourish the skin with natural complements;

    With its natural ingredients, Shea butter provides the skin with natural nutrition. It is a very efficient product to take care of its skin. Indeed, with the various vitamins which compose it, Shea butter is a very effective skin care and protection product. However, in order to benefit from all its virtues, it is advisable to use natural Shea butter.

2. Protect against dry skin;

    Shea butter is a very effective way to get rid of dry skin. It effectively eliminates skin imperfections and helps to guarantee smooth skin.

3.   Hard skin;

Dry skin leads to hard skin. Indeed it is constantly having dry skin that leads to skin imperfection situations. Shea butter feeds the skin. With it, the skin becomes healthy and regains its luster.

4.   Protect from sunburn;

Shea butter is very effective in protecting against UV rays. It is a natural product that has nothing to envy to other products in terms of protection against sunburn.

5.   Prevent skin rashes;

People who use Shea butter are practically free of rash cases. Indeed Shea butter is highly effective in preventing external skin risks. Its nutritional components provide the necessary defensive elements that our skin needs and actively help to nourish and protect it on a daily basis. It is always convenient to use natural products when choosing Shea butter.

Some additional virtues of Shea butter :

o Treat skin cracks;

o To relieve cases of muscle fatigue or muscle pain;

o Treats stains and wrinkles on the skin;

o Treatments for eczema;

o Treating dermatitis;

o Treat small skin wounds.

Conclusion

Conclusion

It was following a personal experience that I decided to write this book in order to share with you the story and bring you with an idea of a natural solution that can help you get rid of this terrible disease which is anal fissure. There are many solutions for treating anal fissures, however, there is not yet one that is 100% guaranteed. Besides, some solutions such as surgery are very expensive, and the results are not yet guaranteed.

With the use of Shea butter, you have a totally natural and very discreet solution. In fact, treating the anal fissure with Shea butter can heal the wound within a few weeks.

Further images of Sea Butter

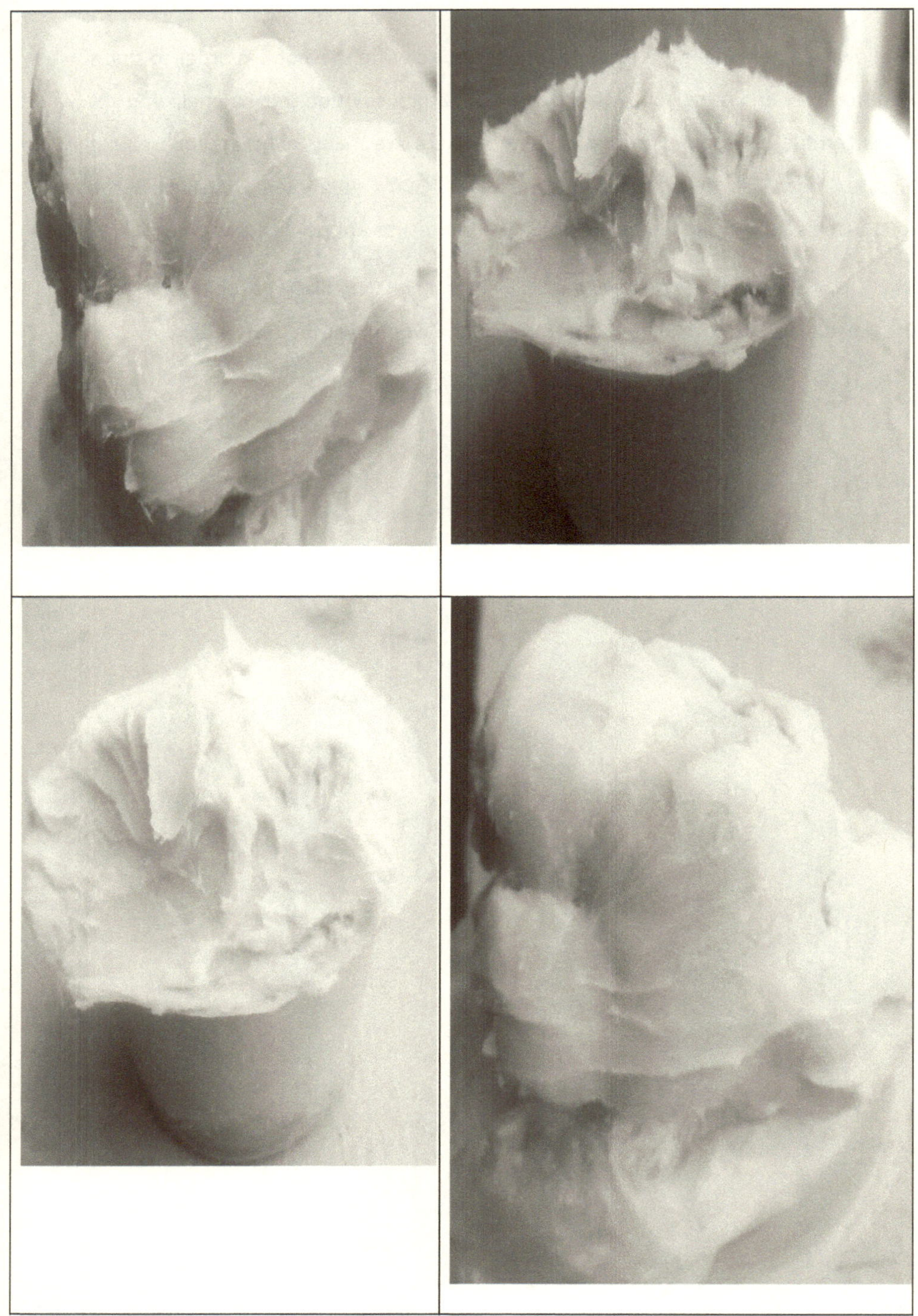

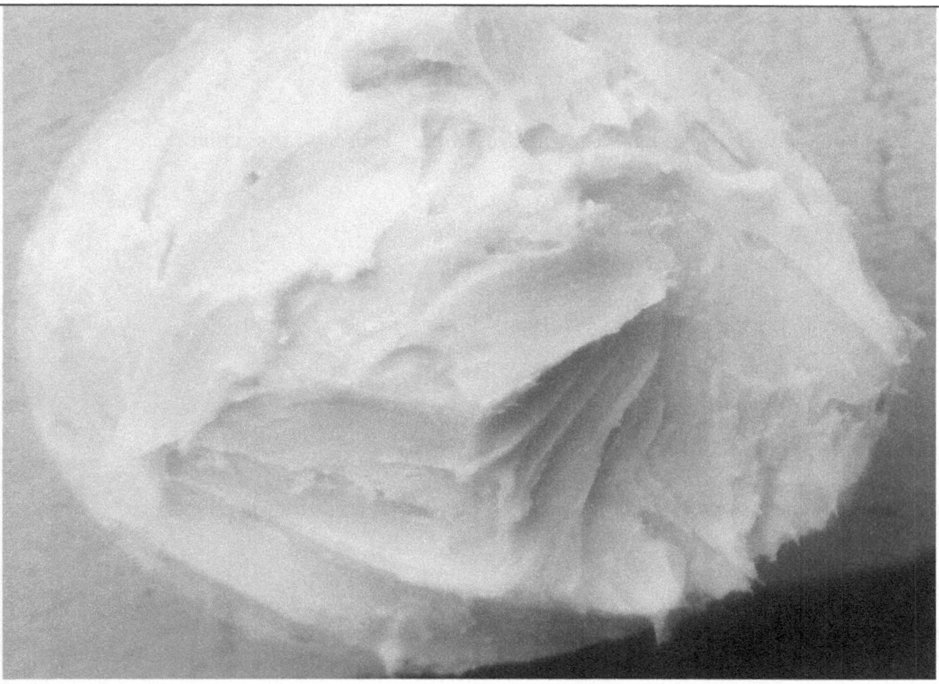

Anal fissure, How to get rid of it naturally and fast

Introduction:

Pains & Issues dealing with the disease. All the stress that it causes to the patient

Chapter 1: What is an anal fissure?

Explanation of what is really anal fissure; - it is anal fissure, no hemorrhoid.

Chapter 2: Causes of anal fissures:

What are the main causes of anal fissures... bad practices that crack the rectal canal...

Chapter 3: The natural and ideal treatment to get rid of anal fissure

The Remedy, the natural product that can help cure fast the disease. Step by step explanation of the procedures.